Squat, Squat, Squat!

How to get a good butt

By:
Christopher Knox

I dedicate this book to my gorgeous koala.
JuliAnee Gutierrez
I love you little one.

Table Of Contents:

Introduction

So you are looking for ways to fix that butt of yours. Maybe you think your butt is flat, maybe you think it is flabby, or maybe you just simply want more muscle to it. In my time as a personal trainer the butt is easily in the top three biggest complaints from women of all ages. Inner thigh fat, under arm flab, belly fat, and the good ol' "i want a better butt."

How do we get ourselves that butt we want to see? Well, I will tell you how. Not only will I give you (list you) many of the best workouts for a great butt and legs that I have come across in my years, but I will also tell you exactly how to perform them and tips to doing them better. Along with providing you things to watch out for.

Now, the book is named 'Squat Squat Squat' but that is only one of the many exercises we will be going over in this book together for our legs and butt. Don't get me wrong though, I am a firm believer in squats and performing your compound movements before all else. Me and thousands of other trainers around the world. Something we DO need to understand and make clear in this book though is that accessory workouts and other compound lifts if provided on the right time scale can absolutely help us further our progression into our final goals.

Without further rambling let's just jump right into the good stuff and start our journey together on the road to a nice butt.

Leg Extension

- The *Leg Extension* is going to be our first leg exercise and will allow you to target your quadriceps which are located in front of your thighs.

- You perform by simply sitting on the bench and by extending your legs up.

- In a machine there will be a pad under your calf and a pad above your shin to keep your leg in place and give you something to push on. Also, the will be a pad above your knees to further keep you in place.

In depth

Leg extensions are looked at by many to be more of a bodybuilding exercise. For our reasons this is fine. I have used them and gotten a lot of return out them for strength as well. For power-lifting they have helped increase my squat. These will be focusing on your legs so you wont really see anything in your butt but you can count on it helping your other lifts improve which will, in turn, help your butt get better.

I use these and I have my clients use these to finish off a good work out a lot of the time. A nice drop set to burn out a great day at the gym is just what you need to have a hard time walking to the locker-room. That extra bit.

Tips

- Try using this as a first exercise and then move to your compound movement. This is called pre-exhaustion and will force your other muscle groups to do most of the work do to your quads already being fatigued.
  - Do NOT always do this. This technique is only to shake things up and shock your muscles.
- Like I said, use this in a drop set at the end of a work out to give yourself that amazing ending you want to feel.

Watch out for

- Try not to over use this exercise. Just like any other exercise you can do it too much so make sure you are mixing up your routine. Otherwise it is a pretty safe workout so have fun.

One-at-a-Time Leg Extension

- The *One-at-a-Time Leg Extension* is a variation on the two legged leg extension exercise.

- It will allow you to target the quadriceps muscles located in front of your thighs.

In depth

Alright, this exercise is just a spin off of the last one. You are just isolating one of your legs. Simple enough right? Clearly you will need to use less weight and focus more. Try to make this one really count. Don't blow this off either just because it seems like less extreme version of the last exercise because this one definitely has it's place.

Tips

- Just do it. Actually do it and don't write it off.

- Provide more focus. While all of your workouts should have a level of focus, give this one some extra TLC and really make sure every rep counts.

Watch out for

- Don't get to excited in these. Be careful and take your time. With one leg you may want to still push the same weight and feel weak if you don't but trust me that will get you nowhere fast. Don't hurt yourself.

Seated Leg Curl

- The *Seated Leg Curl* is similar to the *Leg Extension.* You sit on a bench and move your feet along the pivots formed by your knees.

- However, you push your feet down towards your buttocks and the muscles targeted here are the hamstring muscles, which are located at the back of your thighs.

In depth

Ok, now this is mostly for your hamstrings but it also works your butt. So you could say we are getting into our first butt workout in a way. Hamstrings are very important to us, not only to make us look good, but also to help us stay safe while lifting on a daily basis. If we just do leg extensions and stuff all of the time we will over develop our quads and that is how you pull a hammy. So, in a way this is one of the most important supporting exercises you can perform.

Tips

- This is another one of those supporting workouts that will work great with drop sets and other burn outs to end a workout.

- I love super-setting these with extensions to finish off a workout. It gives each muscle group a small chance to re-coop while you blast the other back to back.

- Try a slower eccentric motion in this lift. (go down slower and control the weight. In other words go slow and make it harder.) This will provide more blood into the myofibrils and even can achieve hyperplasia which will in turn give us bigger stronger muscles.

Watch out for

- You don't really have to watch out for anything special here just grip and rip so to say.

Prone Leg Curl

- The *Prone Leg Curl* is a variation on the *Leg Curl* leg exercise in which you lie prone on a bench instead of being seated.

- The movements are the same in both case, they target your hamstrings equally but sometimes gyms have one type of machines and not the other.

In depth

There is nothing really to in depth to get into with this one other than I like when my girlfriend does these with me. It is self explanatory what the difference is here. All you need to do now is perform! Come on don't make excuses you are a beast and you know you are so go and do it.

Tips

- Try throwing this in a super-set. It work wonders for me and my clients.
- Mix things up by doing some high rep set with this sometimes. Not only will this provide you with a nice burn at the end of your workout but it will also hit a whole different muscle fiber type that you would have not hit otherwise.

Watch out for

- Take it slow. Don't slam and jam out reps like a mad man. Not only is there no reason and taking slow and controlled eccentric movements will build muscle far better but you can EASILY injure yourself doing that in this exercise.

One-at-a-Time Prone Leg Curl

- The *One-at-a-Time Leg Curl* is a close variation where you pull your feet towards your buttocks using one leg at a time.

- It can seem quite stressing on your hamstring muscles to exercise this way but some people find the variation useful.

In depth

Here I another isolated one leg movement. The reason I like these so much is because it really makes you slow down and focus a lot more. Really emphasize that in this exercise. Take up to a five second eccentric motion in this and it will feel amazing.

Tips

- As far as tips go for this one just try adding the 5 second eccentric motion like I mentioned before.
- Also, try throwing in half reps with both the top half and bottom half for added variation.

Watch out for

- This one is a little bit more dangerous especially if you are one of those grunt and groan and slam it around while doing supporting movements people. So just take your time with this one and make sure you are doing it right.

Leg Press

- The *Leg Press* is a leg exercise similar to the squat but where you use gym-type equipment to give resistance to your legs as they are pushing.

- Like the squat, the leg press will develop the muscles located in front of your thighs (quadriceps) and in your buttocks (glutes).

In depth

Ah the leg press. One of my favorites. Even though a lot of my powerlifting buddies hate this and swear it is a bodybuilder workout I think it added loads to my strength. Get deep in these and it will REALLY work that butt. Engaging the glutes is what I aim for in this exercise with female clients most. They come to me asking to improve their butt yet when they gt on the leg press they only go down half way through the rep. Go lower! Get low and don't be afraid. This is one of the best exercises for our butts.

Tips

- Go heavy!
- Do lots of sets and reps. Volume.
- Try different things with this. Go ahead and be creative. Do some wide stance. Do some close stance. Do some with your toes pointed out. Everything has a use, see what works for you.

Watch out for

- Don't flop around in the seat. Keep a steady base and do work.
- Do not let the weight slam down and try to use the momentum for the concentric portion of the lift. You'll gain less muscle and you can easily hurt yourself.

Incline Leg Press

- The *Incline Leg Press* exercise uses a different contraption that puts you in a position to push weight up using your legs.

- This exercise is very popular although special attention needs to be taken so as not to let the weights lower too low to a level where you could become stuck, that is not able to push the weights away.

In depth

Even though this is almost the exact same workout as the last one, this is my favorite of the two. This is what I use most and what I will pick when going between the two. Reason being, it really allows me to get that depth we were talking about that is needed to engage that butt of ours. This one though you do need to be far more careful with than the last one.

Tips

- Again, go heavy!
- This is sort of large movement so it is ok to start with this if you aren't starting with squats or deadlifts.

Watch out for

- Well, everything. This one can be a bit risky. Don't be a show off or think it is helping you to slam the weight off the bottom.
- Try to have a spotter for this one. Especially if you are trying to push yourself or using higher weight than usual.

Squat

- The *Squat* leg exercise uses a gym-type contraption that will allow you to push yourself away like you would in a traditional barbell squat.

- Some machines like the one shown here will have you lying on your back in order to isolate your thighs and glutes.

In depth

Ok, so here we are at the golden lift. The one that is n the title of the book three times. I put this in the middle of the book to make you pay attention and learn some other things and hopefully you did.

So, the squat will be your bread and butter. "When in doubt, squat it out." Just like our other lifts we will need to get depth to make sure we engage our butts. Spread your legs out to about shoulder width or for taller people like me spread them a little wider. Point your toes out ever so slightly. Look up at around a 20 degree angle. Do not cock your head way back and do not look at the ground right in front of you. Now, roll your hips back as if you are about to sit into a chair that has been place directly behind you. Lower, lower, lower till you break parallel and then press back through to the top. Make sure you squeeze your butt on the way up and really engage that portion.

Tips

- This is your compound movement that will help your butt the most so make sure you do your research and do it right.
- Get low!
- Proper form.
- Slow and controlled.
- Go heavy.
- Add volume.

Watch out for

- Have a spotter at all times and if you are going really heavy try getting two side spotters as well.

- Don't cock your head up or look straight down.
- Don't go to fast or bounce up from the bottom like a stripper. I see a lot of girls doing this and it is just wrong. Time under tension is key, especially with this lift.

This is what will help your butt the most. Use it well and use it often. Amen.

Seated Hip Adduction

- The *Seated Hip Adduction* is a great exercise to use if you are looking to strengthen the muscles located in your inner thighs.

- In it you simply try to bring your legs closer to one another by squeezing them together.

In depth

Remember in the beginning when I said that most girls want me to help them with their inner thigh fat? While the fat will come of where it comes off, this will help firm and tone up the area by adding the much needed muscle. All of this plays into getting a better butt believe me. You don't want to have a good butt and flabby inner thighs.

Tips

- As the rock says 'don't look someone in the eyes while you are on this machine.'
- This machine is one that girls will over use. Don't over do it i.e. don't do it every day you go to the gym. Your muscle groups still need that 48 hour minimum window to repair bigger and better than before.

Watch out for

- Nothing really. Just don't look people in the eyes and you are fine.

Standing Hip Adduction

- The *Standing Hip Adduction* is quite similar to its seated variant but will require you to work one leg at a time while you stand on the other.

- It is another great way to strengthen the muscles located in your inner thighs.

In depth

Nothing too out of the ordinary here. Same thing as the last exercise for the most part. This is just another variation so you don't get to use to the same ol' thing. Go ahead, shock your muscles a little bit and change it up.

Tips

- No need to do this so often. The regular movement is spicy enough. This is just if you are feeling bored or prefer it over the later.

Watch out for

- Zombies!
- Make sure you hang on to the handles provided. I took a spill once.

Standing Hip Adduction using Low Pulley

- This variation of the *Hip Adduction* leg exercise uses a low pulley system and requires the same movement of bringing the leg attached to the pulley towards the other.

- You'll again strengthen your inner thigh muscles by using this exercise.

In depth

This movement is actually very cool. I like it do to its unique way of adding the hip adduction movement into your workout. The low pulley gives it a whole new feel. Try it, you might just like it.

Tips

- Try adding more unique ways about attacking certain movements to your workouts just like this does.

Watch out for

- Being to closed minded. I have come across a lot of closed minded people in my years as a trainer and they just don't like the movement from the start. Even though it might work really well for them.

Seated Hip Abduction

- The *Seated Hip Abduction* can be considered the opposite of the *Hip Adduction* exercise.

- In it instead of bringing your legs closer to one another you are pushing them further from each other.

In depth

Now we get into the abduction! How fun is that? Now, in reality this is more of a "butt workout" that the last couple of workouts but like I said before, everything works together to give you the total package. This will work your glute med. It will just add that extra something nice to your butt. You will like it, trust me.

Tips

- Super-set this with the adductors.
- Do higher reps and higher volume sometimes. These muscles will have a different composition than others and may have a higher count of type 2 muscle fibers.

Watch out for

- Forgetting or just not utilizing this tool for your butt arsenal.

Standing Hip Abduction

- The *Standing Hip Abduction* exercise lets you strengthen the muscles located in your hips.

- You perform by pushing the lever outward using your leg that should remain straight throughout.

In depth

This may even be better than the later. In this position you can really get a good contraction and squeeze through that movement all the way from the bottom to the top. That's not even mentioning how it can be used to hold an isometric pause at the top for added muscle growth. Great exercise.

Tips

- Hold at the top for some or all of your reps. Try holding for 2-3 seconds.
- Go slow on the way down. Remember that slow 5 second eccentric motion we talked about earlier? Go ahead.

Watch out for

- Choosing the wrong form of this exercise to fit you. Try them all and see which one fits best.

Standing Hip Abduction using Low Pulley

- Finally the *Standing Hip Abduction on a Low Pulley* exercise lets you strengthen your hip muscles using a low pulley and cable system.

- You perform is as you do other hip abduction exercises by pushing your leg away from the other.

In depth

As with the standing low pulley hip adduction, I really like this one. Not only does it have the brownie points from the last movement but this has the added bonus of its unique nature. Add this for sure into your workouts for a nice butt. It will work nicely.

Tips

- Try this one in a few different ways. Pull it back. Bring your leg forward a little. Variation can't hurt just don't always do it like that is all.

- Here we go again with the amazing isometric opportunity. Amazing is the key word.

Watch out for

- Nothing more than you should watch out for on th last movement. Not much different here.

Calf Raise on Calf Bench

- The *Calf Raise* exercises featured here uses a specially designed bench for calf muscles.

- By putting your toes on the step and pushing the weight pads straight up will target the calf muscles very effectively.

In depth

Let's make sure we don't leave out our calfs. That would just look weird to have a nice butt and nice legs but have small undefined calfs. So lets make a promise right here right now. We will all do calfs. Calf raises are a little different. They are sort of like the biceps of the legs. Some say it is near impossible to over train them. Also, it will help tons if you incorperate higher reps and volume.

Tips

- Add high reps.
- Actually do them!
- High volume

Watch out for

- Neglecting to do them.
- Not adding high rep sets.

Lunges

- The *Lunge* can also be performed using a barbell on your back or dumbbells in your hands.

- You stand up straight and step up and out with one leg. Bend down almost to touching your knee to the ground. Press back up to the starting position all while squeezing your butt tight. Switch legs. Repeat as many times as needed.

In depth

This one is very important and in my opinion should be added quite frequently. I love this exercise. It is wonderful to build your butt and quads. Make sure you get low just like the squats and leg press so you can engage your butt.

Tips

- Get low.
- Squeeze your butt through the top of the rep.
- Add movement into your set. Don't stick to a stand in one pot method or linear walk. Step side to side or even backwards.

Watch out for

- Balance may be an issue. Try holding onto something to start out.

In conclusion

So, to sum this all up. There are lots of ways to make your butt look better and bigger. Squats are our bread and butter so make sure you are doing it right. The butt is a package deal that comes with thighs, hips, calfs, quads, and hammys so don't over do one portion and leave out another part.

Thank you for reading my book. I hope you enjoyed it and learned something. This has been my passion for years and I love nothing more than to see someone learn and better themselves. Meeting goals I a great feeling but helping someone meet their goal is a whole nother ball game. I will have other books and more knowledge to pass on as time goes on.

Go out! Work out! You've got this and I believe in you. Set your goals and shatter them.